HGH GEL

The Anti-Aging Formula for Becoming Younger (The Somatropin Human Growth Hormone)

Copyright 2019 by Michael Joseph - All rights reserved.

This book is geared towards providing precise and reliable information, with regard to the topic and its related topics. This publication is sold with the idea that the publisher is not required to render any accounting, officially or otherwise, or any other qualified services. If further advice is necessary, contacting a legal and/or financial professional is recommended.

-From a Declaration of Principles that was accepted and approved equally by a Committee of the American Bar Association and a Committee of Publishers' Associations.

In no way is it legal to reproduce, duplicate, or transmit any part of this document, either by electronic means, or in printed format. Recording this publication is strictly prohibited, and any storage of this document is not allowed unless with written permission from the publisher. All rights reserved.

The information provided herein is stated to be truthful and consistent, in that any liability, in terms of inattention or otherwise, by any usage or abuse of any policies, processes, or directions contained within, is the solitary and utter responsibility of the recipient reader. Under no circumstances will any legal responsibility or blame be held against the publisher for any reparation, damages, or monetary loss due to the information herein, either directly or indirectly.

Respective authors own all copyrights not held by the publisher.

The information herein is offered for informational purposes solely, and is universally presented as such. The information herein is also presented without contract or any type of guarantee assurance.

The trademarks presented are done so without any consent, and this publication of the trademarks is without permission or backing by the trademark owners. All trademarks and brands within this book are thus for clarifying purposes only and are owned by the owners themselves, and not affiliated otherwise with this document.

Published by Newstone Publishing

ISBN 978-1-989726-13-6 (paperback)

Table of Contents

Introduction	**11**
Disclaimer	**13**
Chapter 1 – Understanding HGH and What It Does For Your Body	**15**
The Basics of HGH	15
What HGH Does For the Body	16
HGH or Somatropin – What's In a Name?	20
The Growth of HGH	21
Chapter 2 – How Much HGH Is In Your Body? (and How Declining Levels Influence Your Body)	**23**
Things That Influence Levels	23
Shifting Changes	25
What Time of Day?	25
Chapter 3 – What Causes Aging?	**27**
Understanding the Four Main Kinds of Aging	27
Lifestyles Can Change	29
Chapter 4 – How HGH Is Produced Within the Body	**32**
The Pituitary Gland	32
Can It Be Removed?	33
How the Hypothalamus Helps	34

Lifetime Points 34

Genetic Factors 35

Three Factors That Influence HGH Release 35

The Concern of Hyper- and Hypo-pituitary Conditions 36

Understanding the Intricacies of HGH 37

Chapter 5 – HGH and Your Immune System 39

Chapter 6 – The Muscle Factor 41

Chapter 7 – Why Your Body Stops Producing HGH (and the Effects) 44

Significant Medical Concerns 45

Chapter 8 – HGH Testing 47

IGF-1 Test 49

Suppression Test 50

Stimulation Test 50

Chapter 9 – Things That Can Mask an HGH Deficiency 52

Chapter 10 – What an HGH Treatment Will Do For You (and What It Won't Do) 54

The Positives of HGH Treatment 54

What HGH Treatment Won't Do 55

What is Hormone Replacement? 57

Chapter 11 – The Hair and Skin Factor 58

Managing Your Hair	58
Working With Skin	59

Chapter 12 – HGH Self-Test   61

When to Self-Test	61
Important Points to Note About Your Body	61

Chapter 13 – The Basics of HGH Gel   64

Why Use a Gel?	64
The General Goal	65
Three Important Ingredients	65
What About Other Ingredients?	66
Identified as Homeopathic	67

Chapter 14 – How Does a Topical HGH Treatment Work?   69

Absorbed by the Skin	69
Targeting the Veins	69
What Makes the Gel Useful?	70

Chapter 15 – Where Does the HGH Come From?   71

How Natural HGH Is Gathered	71
Producing rHGH	72
Controlling the Risk of Creutzfeldt-Jakob Disease	73
The Synthetic Consideration	73

The Development of Somatrem	74
Chapter 16 – How to Get a Prescription For HGH Gel	**75**
Testing Is Required	76
Chapter 17 – How You Should Apply HGH Gel	**77**
How Much Is Needed?	77
Where Is It Applied?	78
The Main Benefit of the Administration Process	78
What About Storage?	79
Chapter 18 – The Use of HGH For Children	**80**
Common Causes and Signs of HGH Deficiency	80
Is the Gel Appropriate For Children?	82
What Inspires People to Get HGH Gel For Their Children?	82
Are There Risks Involved in Using HGH?	83
Chapter 19 – The Dangers of Excess HGH	**85**
Chapter 20 – What Is the Cost?	**88**
Understanding the Expenses For Traditional Treatments	88
How About a Gel Treatment?	88
What About Insurance?	89
A Final Note	**90**

Introduction

Aging is an inevitable thing that comes about in life: problems like sagging skin and looking worn out, losing hair, skin being discolored, and memory issues. Muscle tone can be lost and the added fat around one's body can accumulate. Aging can also change your sexual life.

The fact is that no matter what people do stay healthy and change their lives, they will always age. The changes that can develop will only become worse over time. It is no wonder that so many people spend a lot of money on plastic surgery and other procedures and treatments to mitigate the aging process and they are not always successful.

As unfortunate as it is, everyone struggles with aging issues. We all have hard times managing our bodies. Aging problems are substantial, but it is important to realize you can do something to restore your body. You might find many different supplements that claim to help you deal with aging, but not everything is going to work. As you will see in this guide, there is a useful choice you can utilize when you're aiming to remain healthy while keeping yourself looking good.

There is an option that you can consider for your health right now called HGH or Human Growth Hormone. This is a helpful compound that is naturally produced in your body. However, as you age, your body will stop producing the amount of HGH that your body requires. The good news is that you can restore the HGH levels in your body. HGH works as an anti-aging agent that restores your body and gives you that youthful look that you have always wanted. The power that comes with HGH is something unlike anything you might have ever experienced in your life.

You will learn about many valuable points surrounding HGH, such as how it works, what makes it unique, and how you can restore the HGH in your body.

The details in this guide will help you understand the ingredients in HGH gel and how this compound may work for you. The most important points include understanding where HGH comes from and how it can be used for your daily life. Details on what you should be doing to use the gel are also important as HGH is a sensitive material.

The best part of using HGH is that it is much easier for your body to utilize. The problem with so many treatments is that those solutions aren't necessarily going to take care of the internal issues that cause the body to age. Even surgery that works on the outside of the body will do nothing to manage your hormones. You have to target the issue based on the root cause. This is where an HGH treatment will work for you. The actual restoration of hormones you might be lacking will help you keep feeling and looking healthy.

HGH gel will provide you with the support that you need to feel younger and healthier.

Disclaimer

There are always changes in the medical world that often redefine the things we see and use in our daily lives. As a result, the information in this book, like with any other book about medical concepts, has information that may be subject to change. The producers of this guide cannot be held responsible for the lack of results produced by the product.

Everyone will respond to HGH gel and other HGH treatments differently. There are no guarantees that you will attain the same results through the use of HGH gel as what others may have experienced. Consult your doctor before starting an HGH routine. Your doctor should determine if you are healthy enough to handle an HGH routine or if you need assistance. Your doctor might also have to analyze how well your body is responding to the treatment process.

HGH gel will only be useful if you use it according to your doctor's recommendations. An excess of HGH may be dangerous to your health. Consult a doctor to determine how much HGH is required for your general health. You might have to use a different form of HGH gel depending on what your doctor might suggest.

You are also required to get a prescription for HGH depending on where you are located. Part of this is based on the Crime Control Act of 1990 in the United States, although the laws will vary based on the part of the world that you are in. Acquiring HGH illegally could be interpreted as a crime depending on where you are located.

Be advised that HGH is illegal for use in various athletic competitions. This guide is intended for those who are struggling with HGH levels and need extra help for their daily living needs.

Avoid using HGH if you are attempting to compete in athletic events. Testing processes make it easy for people to identify that someone has been using HGH for any intention.

Chapter 1 – Understanding HGH and What It Does For Your Body

Your body produces many chemicals every day. You might not be aware of it, but your body is very active every day as it produces important compounds needed for your daily health. These include many chemicals that are produced by the brain and various glands. Various signals are sent out to trigger the production of these materials to encourage various actions, behaviors, and other bodily functions. You need those chemicals to help you maintain a healthy body. One such compound that makes a real difference in your life is HGH.

HGH is a compound that dictates how well your body feels, and how young you appear. The problem with HGH is that it is not always going to be there for you because less HGH is produced in your body as you age. A healthy daily routine will entail the addition of extra HGH to assist you with feeling stronger and healthier as you get older.

The Basics of HGH

Human Growth Hormone or HGH is a protein made within the pituitary gland. HGH is also known as somatotropin. The protein specifically works as a peptide hormone. HGH is needed for reproducing cells and to stimulate growth in the body. Much of this includes helping the body to regenerate any cells that might be lost over time.

The best way to describe HGH is that it is a mitogen. That is, it is a chemical compound that triggers cellular division. HGH only targets specific kinds of cells in the body, particularly cells that encourage healthy growth and a proper rate of cellular turnover.

HGH ensures that the body will feel its healthiest while being capable of managing many healthy functions.

HGH is produced within the body through the pituitary gland. The protein is then moved into the bloodstream. The production helps to keep your body active and healthy.

An interesting point about HGH is that it is unclear how much is produced on an average day. HGH tests can reveal different levels of this hormone throughout the day. The production of growth hormones changes at varying points throughout the day, thus making it hard to determine when the body's hormonal levels are at optimum. Regular HGH treatments including HGH gel may make it easier for the body to maintain the proper levels.

HGH is more prominent within the body in childhood. The HGH levels in the body will peak during puberty. Those levels then decline over time. Eventually, the body stops producing the HGH that it needs. You'll learn more about how the rate of HGH production in your body declines later in this book.

It is through HGH that you can maintain a healthy body structure while having the energy you need for doing the things you want to do every day of your life. HGH is also necessary to help you to stay looking young and healthy.

What HGH Does For the Body

HGH is important for the human body in many ways:

1. HGH builds and maintains healthy tissues.

HGH is needed to help the body grow. By producing enough HGH, your body will be restored and healthy. You will feel many benefits when you can stay active and in control. When you feel active, you will have an easier time managing many functions of your body.

2. HGH can improve upon the quality of your skin.

You will look and feel younger when you are producing enough HGH within your body. HGH can slow down the process of aging of your skin cells. This is due to HGH working to enhance your body's cellular turnover rate. By keeping your skin cells restored, your skin will feel healthy and have a look of vitality.

3. Your muscles will become stronger.

You can develop healthier muscles when you use HGH in your regular routine. HGH helps you to build muscle mass. The compound triggers the synthesis of collagen. This important compound is needed to keep the skin and muscle fibers flexible. The skeletal muscles and tendons will become stronger.

This point is a key part of why many patients with HIV and AIDS require HGH treatments. HGH helps to control and slow the muscle wasting process. Although HGH is not a cure for HIV or AIDS, the condition can at least ensure the body will stay healthy longer. This is to keep the progression of the disease from being as intense as it potentially could be.

4. Your body will have an easier time recovering from various injuries.

You can use HGH to help you restore your body tissues following an injury and HGH will improve how well your bones can heal. Much of this is due to HGH assisting in the body's natural production of human growth factors like IGF-1. That particular protein is needed for stimulating healthy bone production. The added support of HGH and the increased cellular production and turnover assists in restoring tissues and helping you heal. You can even use HGH to assist in the healing of bone fractures and other substantial injuries to the body.

5. You may also lose weight when you have enough HGH.

HGH triggers lipolysis in the body. This is the natural breakdown of lipids in the body. Part of this includes having triglycerides converted into free fatty acids. The free fatty acids will be easier to burn off and control within your body. The production of HGH is required to help you with triggering enough fat loss, thus assisting you in losing weight. A lack of HGH will cause your body to lose the effect of lipolysis.

A particularly important aspect of losing weight with HGH is that obese patients often utilize HGH to keep their bodies under control and are less likely to experience added fat gains. Many obese patients have been treated with HGH as part of an extensive weight loss program. Those who have utilized HGH while working with other weight loss efforts lose more on average than others, thus making it easier for people to get more out of their obesity control plans. HGH gel is often utilized in the weight loss process in this case.

6. Your mood may improve after your body takes in HGH.

General studies have found that HGH may assist in improving your mood. Although the effects of HGH will vary according to each person, you may expect to experience enhanced cognitive function and more control over your emotions when you utilize added HGH. You may have an easier time with thinking or making decisions. It should be easier for you to keep yourself focused and in control over your life when you take in enough HGH. In fact, those who take in HGH have reported reduced symptoms of depression.

7. Your sleep will improve over time.

You will experience better sleep when you utilize HGH. Part of this comes as HGH is often influential to how well your body can feel restored. Naturally, you would need to keep your body's HGH stores high enough to keep your body from feeling pains and other problems. The great news is that you will sleep better because you won't struggle with various pains in your body while you're trying to sleep. Another important aspect is that sleep helps you to restore your body's natural HGH production levels, thus giving you extra help with managing how well your body feels.

People who do not get enough sleep will experience a reduced production of natural HGH. This is because the body is unable to handle regular body functions. The lack of sleep keeps your body from feeling restored. The sleep-wake cycle may also change. HGH restores the imbalance in your sleeping routine. This gives you extra control over how well your body feels while ensuring you will not struggle to manage your sleep routine.

8. Your sexual health may also improve.

An attractive benefit of HGH is that this helps improve your sexual health. Much of this comes from your body having more energy. For men, HGH may work even further by stimulating the genital area. This may improve upon how well erections can develop. In addition, the smooth muscles in that area will feel stronger and healthier. This could keep you from developing impotence among other concerns.

9. It may also be easier for your body to make use of the nutrients and vitamins you require.

HGH can help treat short bowel syndrome. This is a condition where the intestine is not functioning properly. Part of this might entail a portion of the intestine having been removed. Those who have short bowel syndrome will be unable to absorb nutrients like vitamins, proteins, fats, and other compounds needed for one's health. Keeping your HGH condition under control will be important to utilize the nutrients. HGH helps to stimulate how well the body can process the nutrients that your body needs for keeping your health in check.

It is exciting to see how well HGH can work for your body. You will need to utilize HGH to help you restore your body and to feel stronger and healthier over time. The design of HGH ensures you'll have more control over your life and feel healthy. However, you must particularly help yourself in getting the most out of your routine when you're aiming to make it easier for your body to stay healthy.

HGH or Somatropin – What's In a Name?

HGH is also referred to by another name called somatropin. Somatropin is the technical or scientific name for HGH. Somatropin is considered to be a recombinant human growth hormone product. The hormone will work with the basic human growth needs that you require including stimulating healthy tissues in the body.

Somatropin takes its name from a growth hormone that is naturally produced by animals and is extracted from their carcasses. This has been often used in many HGH supplements, although some hormones may be extracted from human cadavers. The sourcing used for HGH can vary based on the product you consider, but it helps to see how well this might work for your body and that you have enough control over how well it may work for your body.

Do not assume that somatropin is different from HGH. The two are literally the same. Therefore, you should take a look at any

HGH gel product to see what the ingredients are. When you find somatropin, be assured that you are using a product that will help you with your growth needs.

The Growth of HGH

The most interesting part of HGH is that it is a wonder molecule that has only been growing in popularity as of late. People have started to understand how HGH works and how it can be effective for anyone's life. It was not until recently that people have started to notice what makes HGH an outstanding solution for one's continued health.

HGH has long been gathered from deceased donors. Cadaver brains were utilized to help secrete and produce HGH. While this was an intriguing solution for gathering HGH and continues to be utilized in some parts of the world, it has become mostly obsolete. It was determined that some people might be at risk of serious medical issues caused by the use of HGH from cadavers. It was not until the 1980s that people started to notice something intriguing and unique with regards to the production of HGH. HGH can be produced by a more acceptable approach.

A 1990 report in the New England Journal of Medicine revealed an amazing story that helped to show just how valuable HGH can be and that the hormone is nowhere near as difficult for people to find or obtain as they once thought. The prominent journal reported on how a synthetic form of HGH was produced. Also known as rHGH, the tissue was found to help many people restore their bodies. People who had dealt with difficult fat deposits and a lack of muscle mass were starting to get their natural body shapes back again. People with gray hair were getting back to their natural hair colors once more. There was also the benefit of people developing healthier bodies following the consumption of HGH.

The general analysis of those who had been using HGH in the test also found that many organs were capable of re-growth. This included the organs returning to their regular sizes and function.

Additional details on how HGH gel is produced will be explained later in this book. This includes looking at how the synthetic form is produced and why that option is much better and safer than the old version that had been gathered from human cadaver donors. HGH can help keep you feeling younger and healthier. You'll have to see for yourself how well this can work for you to stay healthy and feel younger.

Chapter 2 – How Much HGH Is In Your Body? (and How Declining Levels Influence Your Body)

An HGH test, which will be discussed later, will help you identify how well your body is handling HGH. You must be aware of how the levels of this hormone in your body can shift over time. The changes in HGH levels might be dramatic.

Your HGH levels will be measured in ng/ml or nanograms per milliliter. This is a measure of your blood based on how much of the hormone is found in a small amount of blood. The HGH in your body, like other things that enter your blood, may be minimal in quantity and yet can make a world of difference.

The average HGH level in a healthy person will vary by age and gender. For men, a person should have fewer than 5 ng/mL of HGH. A woman should have less than 10 ng/mL of HGH. A child would have up to 20 ng/mL of HGH with that total peaking at puberty. These values are relative to individual people and can show how the body is producing its HGH levels. Any case where the body is producing less than or more than what is necessary could be a threat to the body as it suggests the body is not getting enough of the HGH that it requires for optimum health.

Things That Influence Levels

Sometimes you might go through certain behaviors or activities that will cause the level of HGH to change. A good example of this is how the hormones might become elevated based on what you are doing, your diet, and your physical routine.

1. Fasting

Fasting is a process where you abstain from food for a certain period of time. Your body's HGH levels will rise when you are fasting. These levels may increase to where you are producing more of the hormone than necessary. Fasting will cause the HGH to elevate to help you reduce the fat stored in your body.

HGH encourages the production of healthy muscle tissue. At the same time, HGH may also regular how much fat is produced and stored. An elevated HGH level during the fasting process will increase the hormone's ability to break down the fatty tissues in your body. The lipolysis effect will release fatty acids and glycerol. These are then processed by the body to produce energy. It takes a while for the HGH to rise during the fasting process. It can take about 12 hours or more for the HGH levels in your body to rise and work a little harder.

Not having enough HGH can be a problem. You might start fasting when you are older, but the HGH you have will not be as effective. The HGH will not be as prevalent in the fasting effort, thus causing the loss of proteins in your muscles to increase. You're not actually going through lipolysis at this point. Instead, your body is utilizing its proteins to keep fats off. This is why you're going to lose muscle mass over time; your body is not able to handle the fats correctly.

2. Stress

Another thing that may influence your HGH totals is stress. The growth hormones in your body will increase when your body notices it is going through stressful situations. This includes concerns where you might be forced into more work than what you can handle. The emotional and physical stress involved can be intense. A drop in HGH levels will cause you to experience more fatigue, thus keeping you from being able to handle all the stress in your life as well as you might wish you could.

3. Exercise

Exercise is important for your daily life and HGH in your body is responsible for helping you to stay active and to keep your muscles functioning during a workout. The lack of HGH as you age can make your muscles weaker and not easy to restore themselves due to not having enough HGH to repair the tissues. This will make it harder for you to stay active and functional in your workouts.

Shifting Changes

One thing to note about HGH levels is that it can be hard to determine how much HGH you have with only one review. The HGH levels in your body will change throughout the day.

You can have an HGH test to see how well you are producing this compound in your body.

The reason why HGH levels change so much is that your pituitary gland releases HGH in pulses. It is difficult to determine precisely when your gland is working with only one blood test. As a result, you would have to have several blood tests to identify how well you are producing HGH. The tests may review if you are going through elevated or regular idle levels. Even then, the shifts may identify times when you are not getting enough HGH. The testing process might entail getting blood drawn every two hours over the course of one day.

What Time of Day?

HGH levels are more prominent in the morning hours than during at any other time of the day. As a result, a testing process will have to take place during the afternoon or evening hours to get a better idea of how well your body naturally produces HGH.

The pulses that your pituitary gland produces with will vary based on the time of day. It is not necessarily easy to predict when those pulses are going to happen. You can expect those pulses to be more prevalent during the earliest hours of the day.

You can talk with a doctor about getting tested to see how well your body is producing HGH. The testing effort should help identify how well your body uses HGH. Remember that any case where you have less HGH than needed will be a sign that you will need some extra help with getting your HGH totals in check. This includes working with a suitable HGH gel treatment to keep your body healthy.

Chapter 3 – What Causes Aging?

No one likes to accept aging. Aging is a fact of life and can be demoralizing to some people. You might get smarter and wiser with years, but that does not mean your body is going to be any better. The interesting thing about aging is that it is an issue that can come along in many forms and can be frustrating for anyone to live with. Let's look at what causes aging and how this concern impacts the body.

Understanding the Four Main Kinds of Aging

Aging is a process that entails more than just your body looking older or you are possibly as active as you used to. Aging also involves how your body changes over the years in many forms. You may go through cellular, metabolic, hormonal, or accumulated aging depending on your body type and what you subject yourself to over time.

1. Cellular

The first form of aging is changes in your cells. Cells are capable of replicating themselves many times. As your cells die, they are replicated by new cells taking their place. Those cells can only do that so many times before they stop altogether. On average, your cells can reproduce about 50 times before they die and no longer reproduce. Much of this is due to those cells changing in texture and no longer forming properly. Part of this is due to the addition of free radicals in your body. The cells that have to be multiplied can be a concern as your body may struggle to replace every one of those cells.

The telomeres in the cells are important to cellular aging. Telomeres are located at the ends of the chromosomes in the cells. These telomeres are critical for maintaining the chromosomes. When a cell divides, the telomeres are not duplicated like the DNA is. This keeps the telomeres from being as functional as they should be. Those parts will get smaller every time a cell is reproduced. The integrity of the cell is minimized due to the telomeres weakening, thus becoming harder on the body.

Cellular aging is the most prominent part of what causes you to look older. As you go through cellular aging, you will experience issues in your body ranging from added wrinkles to age spots and other things. All of those dead skin cells will add up over time and become very hard to manage

2. Hormonal

Hormonal aging occurs when the hormone levels in your body shift and decrease. Hormonal changes cause dry skin and menopause among other issues. Much of this is due to the body's endocrine system not being as effective as it used to be. The endocrine system is responsible for producing the key hormones needed for reproduction, growth, and other vital functions in the body. The changes will cause you to age sooner.

Naturally, HGH is one of the hormones that will be impacted the most by the endocrine system not being very effective. IGF-1, a growth factor, may also be impacted. The levels of HGH and IGF-1 among other growth-related hormones might be inconsistent. It will be harder for your body to grow properly and to look its youngest due to this concern.

3. Metabolic

Metabolic aging is a threat that occurs from the byproduct of metabolic processes within the body. Your cells are responsible for converting foods to energy. The byproducts generated in the metabolic efforts can be harmful and cause premature aging.

This has led to some believing that restricting one's calories and slowing down metabolic processes may be recommended.

The rate of living theory states that those who metabolize oxygen and other compounds faster will have shorter life spans. For instance, smaller mammals that have fast heartbeats do not live as long because they utilize oxygen quickly. A turtle will live for a hundred years or longer because that mammal does not process oxygen as fast as others. This leads to the belief that those who can handle metabolic processes slowly will live longer. This may be relevant to one's appearance and physical performance, although it can be difficult to control when a strong effort to consume foods is considered.

4. Accumulation

The accumulation that develops in the body comes from outside sources. You may be exposed to various toxins, pollutants, dangerous foods, smoke from cigarettes, and many other things that you might be exposed to. Outside elements can damage your tissues. The body will not be able to repair or maintain its cells as well as it should. The threat can be dangerous and problematic in many cases, thus making it harder for the body to be functional.

All people will experience these forms of aging. The good news is that HGH treatments can help with restoring many parts of the body while working to counter all of these forms of aging. HGH will help you look and feel younger, but it may also improve your physical performance.

Lifestyles Can Change

Your lifestyle may be a consideration that makes it harder for you to age naturally and make you age prematurely. Let's look at some of the ways how your lifestyle might be a factor in aging.

1. You might not be eating healthy.

Your diet may be a factor as to why you are not aging well. It is increasingly difficult for people these days to eat healthily. With so many sugars, salts, artificial ingredients in our foods, it is difficult to find things that are suitable to eat. Choosing only healthy foods may also be too expensive and restrictive. It is hard for people to find foods that are suitable for many dietary demands because of this.

2. Smoking is a problem.

Even though there are so many restrictions on where people can and cannot smoke, it is still easy to come across smoke in many forms. Smoking is prevalent throughout the world. You might struggle to avoid it altogether. You have to stop smoking if you already do so. However, it might take a while or be impossible to reverse the effects of smoking.

3. You might not be getting enough exercise.

It is easy to skip exercising. Our lives are so busy these days that it is next to impossible for us to stay active and in control of our lives. Getting 15 to 30 minutes of exercise a day for five days in a week should help you to stay healthy and in control of your body. Even then, it might be a challenge for you to try and get all that exercise to work for you. You might be too tired from all that work you put into your daily routine. Then again, fatigue is a commonplace sign of aging and can be a burden to your life.

4. You aren't getting the sleep you require.

People often do what they can to try to get more work done while not getting enough sleep. However, sleep is necessary for reducing stress levels and for allowing the body to restore its natural functions. Not getting enough sleep will make it difficult for your body and your brain to stay active and sharp.

    5.   Stress makes life harder for everyone.

Stress can be a burden to anyone's life, but it is a problem that can make it easier for your body to age faster than normal. Stress makes it harder for you to focus and to keep your body healthy. More importantly, your body might struggle to keep up with everything that's happening, thus causing intense fatigue. Keeping stress in your life in check is important for a healthy life.

HGH treatments may help reduce some of the effects of aging.

Chapter 4 – How HGH Is Produced Within the Body

HGH is a necessity for keeping you from aging. HGH is naturally produced in your body, but the amount produced decreases with age. It might be difficult for your body to produce the HGH that it needs. Outside support may be required for you to get HGH to work to your benefit.

Your brain is responsible for the production of HGH. It is through the glands and other parts of your brain that various chemicals and neurotransmitters are produced. You can utilize HGH to help you restore your brain's functions and to stay active and alert. There may be times when your body does not have the support from glands to produce the HGH that you require for your health.

The Pituitary Gland

The pituitary gland is the most important part of the HGH production process. The gland is small in size and is located in the middle part of the brain. It is near the base and is directly under the hypothalamus. The gland is often referred to as the master gland as it produces hormones that are needed for restoring the body's natural functions. This may also stimulate other nearby glands to help produce other healthy hormones.

The pituitary gland is responsible for releasing HGH into your body and works at various intervals or bursts. The gland will produce the hormone every three to five hours on average. The effort moves the hormone into the bloodstream to allow the body to use it.

The gland may be damaged over time for many reasons. Sometimes it might be damaged due to a tumor or other problems. A tumor might limit the production of HGH or may also produce an excess. In other cases, the gland might not be getting a large enough blood flow.

This gland is vital for more than just helping you to take care of how growth hormones are produced. The gland is also responsible for the production of ACTH, a hormone that stimulates the adrenal glands and helps them to release cortisol, a compound that regulates the body's blood pressure and metabolic rate. The pituitary gland also triggers the production of healthy thyroid hormones. Follicle-stimulating hormones are also supported trigger sexual functions in one's body. The gland is also critical for women in that it helps in the production of prolactin, a hormone needed for the stimulation of milk production and the growth of female breasts.

It should also be noted that the pituitary gland regulates the production of the melanocyte-stimulating hormone. This is a hormone that is responsible for regulating skin pigmentation. Any changes in how the gland is working might be noticed by the skin looking discolored in some way. The skin could either appear darker or lighter than usual. This could be another sign that you have issues with your pituitary gland.

Each of these points relating to the gland is vital to its operation. You might begin to notice something is off if any part of your body is not working as well as it needs to.

Can It Be Removed?

One of the most common issues surrounding the pituitary gland is that the organ may be removed. There are times when the pituitary gland has to be removed from the brain. These are typically for cases when there are tumors or other significant growths that can cause an improper amount of HGH to develop. In other cases, there might be some cancerous growth on the organ that requires the gland to be removed.

A transsphenoidal surgery occurs when the pituitary gland is removed. The process is done to get rid of the unhealthy tumor without impacting the rest of the brain. While this helps eliminate the unhealthy area, this will stop the body from producing HGH. The patient would require regular HGH treatments throughout their life to respond to the body's inability to naturally produce the hormone. As difficult as this may be for many people, the surgical procedure is an unfortunate necessity that has to be carried out.

How the Hypothalamus Helps

The hypothalamus is important in the HGH production process. This is in the middle part of the brain that influences the release of hormones. The hypothalamus is needed to stimulate the pituitary gland to help release the growth hormone as needed. Somatostatin may also be produced in the effort to inhibit the release of the hormone when needed. The hypothalamus produces that compound to ensure that the HGH is released within the right time for the best results.

Lifetime Points

The HGH hormone may be produced at greater amounts depending on the time in one's life. Specifically, HGH is produced at its greatest rate in puberty and childhood until the child grows to adult size. The HGH production levels should decline after puberty and will continue to narrow over time.

HGH production is reduced dramatically during pregnancy. A woman who is pregnant will not produce HGH as much due to the brain noting that such growth factors are already high in the bloodstream. Those growth factors are working within the body to support the unborn child.

Genetic Factors

The body's genes may also be factors that will directly influence how HGH is produced. The q22-24 region of chromosome 17 has been found to be influential to how HGH can be produced. The growth hormones that may be produced are located in this part of the chromosome. Genetic testing may identify how HGH is produced. People who have deficiencies in those parts of their chromosomes may be at a higher risk of growth-related problems, although it might be easier for those issues to develop at a younger age.

Three Factors That Influence HGH Release

There are three factors that will directly influence how well you can handle HGH, but they are also points that can become less intensive and less powerful as you age.

1. Growth hormone releasing hormone

There is a hormone that is needed within the body to help release HGH. The growth hormone releasing hormone or GHRH is a compound that triggers the pituitary gland's functionality. This regulates the gland into releasing more HGH over time. Your body will be depleted of GHRH after a certain time. This hormone is most prominent in puberty.

2. Growth hormone releasing peptide

The GHRP is a peptide that also declines with age. This is also responsible for telling the pituitary gland to restore its production of HGH.

3. Somatostatin

Somatostatin is a hormone that regulates how much HGH is produced within the body. This keeps your body from making more HGH than what you can handle. The hormone will block the pituitary gland from producing increased amounts of HGH. Somatostatin can help keep your body protected from excess HGH and there will be an overall decline in HGH production over the years.

The Concern of Hyper- and Hypo-pituitary Conditions

Not all people have pituitary glands that are healthy enough to handle HGH well. Some people may experience hyper-pituitary or hypo-pituitary conditions. These are respective conditions where the body makes more or less HGH than necessary. The conditions are difficult and they can become extremely intense.

A gland that produces excess HGH will promote gigantism and other problems that might encourage excessive growth. This would require the gland to be removed. A gland that does not produce enough HGH will not have to be removed, but the person who has that condition would require HGH supplementation over time. Either way, any person with a gland that does not work properly would require extra HGH, particularly HGH gel. The question is whether or not the gland in question has to be removed. Naturally, an overactive gland would need to be removed.

For a weak gland, some medications may be used to try to get the gland to start functioning and to stay active. In many cases, an outside HGH gel compound may be required for treatment. Only a doctor can say for certain what you need to use to take care of the condition.

Understanding the Intricacies of HGH

Although HGH is a vital part of the body's natural functionality, it is not necessarily a point that has been studied intensely. HGH was first identified by the National Institute of Health in the mid-twentieth century. The discovery of HGH was critical to identify how the body grows.

HGH functions for the most part as an anabolic. That is, the compound will build up muscle mass and other tissues, thus helping you stay active. Growth hormone works as a material that can receive certain cells of value to you. The hormone will bind to the receptors of target cells around your body. Such cells may be found around the muscle tissues, and many are found in the liver.

The HGH compounds will move around target cells. The growth hormone is unable to penetrate cell membranes. This is due to the hormones not being fat-soluble. The effects will be produced by binding to the receptors found on target cells. A series of proteins will interact with the cells to trigger certain functions. Specifically, the MAPK/ERK pathway will be utilized in the process. This pathway is responsible for stimulating the division of muscle cells. The healthy production of new cells makes it easier for the body to produce enough cells and make the area healthy.

The growth hormone that moves into the liver will trigger the production of IGF-1. This is insulin-like growth factor 1, a hormone that has a molecular body similar to that of insulin. This offers an anabolic effect and may help control issues relating to growth failure in the body. The compound helps to restore a healthy body structure and improves how well the tissues feel and function.

HGH is frequently recognized as being important for children who are growing and will also improve many other functions. Your muscle mass will increase through hypertrophy, a process that entails the body taking in more hormones and becoming stronger.

Many other things will be noticed within your body as you use HGH:

1. The proteins in your body will be easier to process. They will synthesize rather quickly.

2. Lipolysis, a process that entails the body burning off fats, will be increased over time.

3. The liver will have an easier time processing glucose. The risk of the liver not being as functional will be minimal.

4. The immune system will be stimulated and active.

5. You should experience a slightly enhanced sex drive.

The outstanding nature of HGH makes it a popular hormone to include in your life. Having a way to restore that HGH in your body is important because your body will stop producing HGH on its own as years go by. This can be a frustrating concern and it can be frustrating to bear with problems relating to the loss of HGH. HGH gel can help you restore what you have lost so it may be easier for you to get the most out of your body.

Chapter 5 – HGH and Your Immune System

You might have heard stories over the years about how your immune system plays a huge role in your life. It is through the immune system that you can fend off many illnesses and other concerns that keep you from staying active. You don't have to live with a weakened immune system forever. HGH can do more for your body and your immune system when all is considered.

As you age, your immune system will start to lose effectiveness. The immune system is responsible for helping your body to fend off illnesses and other medical concerns. You will need the white blood cells and T-cells that make up the immune system to help keep foreign bodies from attacking or influencing your body negatively. You can utilize those immunity-producing bodies to help you keep your body from feeling excess fatigue. There is also a potential for the body to look healthier too because of the cells clearing out old skin cells that might not be as healthy as they should be.

HGH has been found in various studies to help with restoring many parts of your body, but it is your immune system that might benefit the most from an HGH treatment. Much of this can be noticed when HGH has been used on people who have immune deficiencies. Specifically, it has been given to people who have HIV and AIDS, two conditions that are prominently recognized by immune deficiencies. People with such conditions have been using HGH for years to control the effects of muscle wasting, one of the most prominent signs of HIV and AIDS. A review in 2002 found that HGH can do more than just that.

The 2002 XIV International AIDS Conference was held in Barcelona to highlight understanding how AIDS may be controlled and what can be done to help the lives of those who have been impacted by AIDS. A review that was presented at the Barcelona event found that HGH can produce a positive impact on the thymus, a lymph organ near the upper breastbone. It is through the thymus that T-cells that make up the immune system can mature. In addition, white blood cells will detect the difference between healthy cells and unhealthy ones. The T-cells may be reviewed by the white blood cells to be antigens that stimulate immune system responses.

People with AIDS were given about 4 mg of HGH per day during the treatment process. Almost all of the people experienced noticeable increases in CD4 and CD8 cell counts. This means that the body will not produce as many unhealthy cells. The body will handle healthier immune system cells and will have strong thymic functions. The addition of HGH helped to ensure that the immune system would be stronger while also distinguishing between different functions of the body.

So, how does this discovery relate to you? This discovery shows that it will be easier for the body's immune system to stay active when you have enough HGH to work with. The body will feel restored and capable of acting properly. More importantly, you will find it is not hard for you to stay focused. You need to have a healthy immune system if you are going to get a good daily routine going. That immune system is vital for helping you to feel restored and positive. You can use HGH to help you with growing and becoming healthier while keeping your immune system under control.

Chapter 6 – The Muscle Factor

Your muscles are important for helping you to look younger. You need muscle mass to look and feel your best while having a younger appearance. The problem is that the aging process makes it harder for your muscles to develop and feel their best. Fortunately, the human growth hormone helps you to keep your muscles strong and healthy.

How is HGH going to help you build muscle mass? Many athletes have tried to use HGH for getting greater muscle mass, even it if is illegal for them to do it this way. The main thing about building muscle mass with HGH is that the compound will help you to burn off fat. HGH does more than just trigger lipolysis. HGH will also influence how well your body can manage the production of healthy muscle fibers and cells while keeping your muscles strong.

Your body's muscle fibers will weaken with age. Eventually, your body will become weaker and it becomes easier for your body to store fats as you age. These points may be noticed in many people who are older in age, but those problems will be even more pronounced in those who have muscle wasting-related conditions, particularly HIV and AIDS.

Over time, your body will start to develop higher blood lipid totals. This entails your blood having more fat in its content. Meanwhile, you may also resist insulin at a greater rate. This means that you might be at risk of storing more fat, thus making it harder for you to naturally use your muscle fibers. These problems keep your muscles from being as useful and productive as they should be. Even worse, those muscles will not be as firm or powerful as you might wish they could be, thus leading to a sizable problem within your body.

HGH will trigger the healthy production of new muscles by helping you with the lipolysis process. The visceral adipose tissue or VAT in your body will decline. This abdominal fat will become easy to burn off.

The Focus of Sarcomere Hypertrophy

Sarcomere hypertrophy is the process of the development of healthier and larger muscle fibers around the body, thus helping you to look younger while that body fat will be less visible. What causes hypertrophy to develop, and what does this entail in general? It becomes easier for your body to handle natural muscle growth when HGH is included in your routine.

The main part of hypertrophy is that the sarcomeres are influenced. A sarcomere is a unit of muscle tissue. The tissue can form the skeletal muscles and will directly influence how well the muscle mass around the body can be formed. Hypertrophy triggers the sarcomeres and allows them to stay active.

HGH triggers the hypertrophy process. The compound allows for the production of new cells around the sarcomeres. Those added muscle cells help produce muscular bulk and strength.

As the muscle cells grow, the muscles are capable of handling more weight. They can also work with greater resistance levels. The most important part of the muscle cells is that they will feel strong enough to recover from even the most difficult forms of pressure. The risk of muscles tearing or prematurely wearing out will be minimal when enough HGH is incorporated in your routine.

For this to work, it is important for you to look at how well your body can manage and use HGH. You will need to use HGH alongside a healthy diet and exercise routine for you to get the best results. This includes being aware of how your body handles the nutrients needed for growing muscle mass while also triggering enough functions within the muscles.

Building muscle mass while adding HGH to your routine will help you look and feel younger.

Chapter 7 – Why Your Body Stops Producing HGH (and the Effects)

The greatest concern surrounding HGH and your body is that you are at risk of losing HGH over time. Specifically, your body will not produce HGH as well as it did when you were younger.

The main reason why your body stops producing HGH is that the brain determines if there is enough HGH in the bloodstream. You will start to experience a drop in HGH production as you reach the age of 30 on average.

Your pituitary gland will have been most active during puberty. The gland will notice that your body does not have enough HGH, thus allowing for added production during this point in life. When you reach the age of 30, your HGH levels will be about a fifth of what they were when you were younger. Your HGH levels will eventually decline by about 10 to 15% every ten years on average. While you might never lose all of your HGH, the effectiveness of that hormone will have weakened to the point where the hormone is not as effective as it should be.

Decreased level of HGH is not the only cause of aging. HGH may help you to stay active longer and in control of your body. You might not be producing as much of this hormone as you might wish you could, thus making it harder for your body to manage its natural functions.

Your pituitary gland might stop working as well over time. The gland might not be active enough or capable of producing enough hormones to stay active. The lack of production may hurt your body and make it difficult for you to manage some of your regular routines. The lack of support from your gland will keep you from feeling healthy and active.

Significant Medical Concerns

A lack of HGH can cause the development of major medical issues that can influence how well you feel. You may experience problems following the lack of HGH in your body, although those issues can be influenced by many outside factors.

1. Your fat mass may increase.

Not having enough HGH may make it harder for you to get the lean body mass you desire. As your body struggles to manage natural metabolic efforts, it becomes easier for you to develop more body fat. This includes fat that develops around the midsection. These fat deposits are often the hardest for you to eliminate. It may also be harder for you to burn off that fat because you are not being as active.

2. You will have less muscle mass.

Your muscle mass could be a factor that will influence your body and how functional it is. You will lose muscle mass over time due to your body not having enough HGH. You need that growth hormone to help improve your workouts and how healthy you can keep your body. This is why so many athletes attempt to break the rules of competition by taking HGH supplements.

3. You may develop an excessive amount of intracellular fluid.

The fluid, in this case, refers to the added fluids that collect outside of the cells in your body. The metabolic efforts that work within your body might be more intense than they should be. The added fluid will make it harder for your body to process many of its functions and to stay as active as it should be.

4. Lability is a problem that results in sudden changes in your mood.

A lack of energy is one problem that you might have when you do not get enough HGH, but lability can be just as difficult to manage. You may experience lability when you experience changes in your mood. Sometimes you might not feel motivated. You might feel tired suddenly without much warning. Depression may also be a problem related to lability in many people.

5. Your cognitive functions will be impaired.

The dreaded brain fog is a problem that can influence your life in many ways. Having little HGH impacts and impairs the brain. The changes may be too dramatic and can cause some sizable shifts in your emotional functionality. This is a concern that might make it harder for you to stay focused at your workplace and make it harder to make rational decisions.

The threat of not having enough HGH in your body is significant. You could be at risk of serious health issues if you do not have the HGH you need. The good news is that you can get tested to see how much HGH you have in your body. The next chapter is all about understanding how testing work and what you can learn from them.

Chapter 8 – HGH Testing

A quick note: HGH testing is designed mainly to identify pituitary problems. This includes a review of cases of stunted growth or gigantism among others. The testing process is not routine, as it is mainly for extreme conditions.

HGH levels can change quite a lot throughout the day. It might be difficult to notice how these levels shift. Review your HGH totals based on what is appropriate for your life. You can talk with a doctor to determine the correct HGH levels for your lifestyle.

You will need to undergo an HGH test to confirm how well your body can take in HGH. You can use an HGH test to confirm if you need an HGH gel treatment.

The HGH serum test is the general test that is used to see how well your body is using the compound. This test is for general low-HGH reviews to see if there are problems in your body about how HGH is developing and being used. The test has also been used by various sporting organizations, particularly the National Football League and International Olympic Committee to identify cases of athletes abusing HGH as a means of getting an advantage over other competitors.

The process can take a while to complete. This is due to the HGH production effort in your body is always inconsistent. You need to get enough reviews of your blood to identify how well you are producing the HGH that you need. This may take a few samples and can work for a few hours at a time. The test is necessary when you have a plan in mind for making your efforts useful.

The good news about the HGH test is that it does not take much effort. It requires the following steps:

1. You will have to fast for at least 12 hours prior to the test.

Basic fasting ensures that your body will not be influenced by any outside compounds. Anything you consume might influence the results of a test. This includes cases where blood sugar levels might change or shift. You should be allowed to drink water before the test as a means of staying hydrated. Anything that might include flavorings or other outside features might influence blood sugar levels, thus influencing the test.

2. Avoid biotin consumption for at least 72 hours prior to the test.

Biotin is a vitamin that improves the health of your hair, skin, nails, and other key parts of your body. Biotin is vital for helping you to keep your body growing well and for handling metabolic processes. This could influence the results of an HGH test. You must avoid consuming biotin in any form especially supplements for at least 72 hours.

3. The timing of the test should be considered.

You need to consider when you're going to complete the HGH test. As mentioned earlier, HGH levels are naturally elevated in the morning. Therefore, you should schedule a test later in the day for the best and most accurate results.

4. A blood test is required.

A doctor may take two separate blood samples to see how well your body is taking in HGH. A third might be required in some cases, although unlikely.

5. You will need to rest for about 30 minutes after the blood test is completed.

Resting after the blood is taken ensures that the blood sample that was gathered is secure. You should not have to worry about experiencing an intense amount of fatigue following the test, although the way a person responds will vary.

6. The test results should be ready in about two to three days.

The readout should include a listing of how well your body is using and producing HGH.

IGF-1 Test

An IGF-1 test may also be conducted alongside a review of your HGH levels. The problem with a standard HGH test is that your body's HGH levels will shift throughout the day. There's a chance that you might not have a high HGH readout even if you are regularly producing HGH. Therefore, an IGF-1 test will be required. Your levels of Insulin Growth Factor-1 may determine whether or not you are producing enough HGH in your body. When you have a higher or lower than average total of HGH, you are also producing an equally higher or lower IGF-1 total.

The IGF-1 test can be handled during the same blood test as your HGH review. The effort for preparing for the test and the process of drawing blood itself will remain the same. The results can also be produced at the same time as the HGH results. Therefore, the IGF-1 test will help ensure that the results of your HGH review are accurate and sensible.

IGF-1 levels will remain stable throughout the day. This is different from the HGH levels which fluctuate during the day.

Suppression Test

The suppression test is used to determine if you are producing more HGH than necessary. The test is important because producing an excessive amount of HGH may be risky to your body. An excess amount might cause significant delays in how HGH is produced at certain times and at other times it will spike. This creates an inconsistent flow of HGH that might not be easy to handle. The test requires a few extra steps for its support.

First, a doctor or nurse will have to take a blood sample. After this, you would consume a particular solution that contains glucose, a common type of sugar. A few more samples of blood would then be drawn over a two-hour period. The samples are taken at various times to identify how well your body is producing HGH with the total value varying.

In most cases, glucose will lower HGH production. Your hormone levels will be checked to see how they are changing following the consumption of the glucose solution. A normal test result would be below 0.3 ng/mL and this suggests that you are producing a normal amount of HGH. Anything that might be outside of that range could be a sign that you have too much HGH and that the HGH gel treatment may be too risky for you.

Stimulation Test

A stimulation test requires that you provide a blood sample and then take a medication that triggers your body to release HGH. The professional should monitor your reaction to the test. A few additional test samples will take place over the next two hours. The samples are then tested to see how well your body is producing HGH.

A stimulation test should result in a reading of 4 ng/mL for adults. For children, that reading should be 5 ng/mL.

By reviewing the results of the testing, it can be determined your body's HGH levels and if you do require any form of HGH treatment. Your doctor will give you advice as to whether or not you could benefit from HGH treatments.

Chapter 9 – Things That Can Mask an HGH Deficiency

It is imperative for you to be tested to see how well your body is producing HGH and that you have enough of this hormone. There is a potential that your body might be dealing with other concerns in your life that are keeping you from noticing that you have low HGH. The symptoms of HGH may be masked by many outside concerns that can influence how well you feel. You might require some extra testing to see if these problems are prevalent. Added tests may be needed in addition to reviews about how well your body is producing HGH.

1. Excess amounts of testosterone

Testosterone is needed for the body to stay active and functional. Testosterone levels can increase over time, thus making it easier for the body to stay active. An elevated testosterone level may mask the lack of HGH in your body.

2. Thyroxin levels.

Thyroxin is a hormone that is produced by the thyroid gland. The hormone is needed to support the natural functionality of your heart and your digestive system. An excess amount of this hormone may hide the fact that you have HGH-related problems within your body. A test may be conducted to see how well your body is producing thyroxin.

3. Cortisol deficiencies

Your body naturally produces cortisol as a response to stress and fatigue. The hormone is not something that people can control, but it is a concern that directly influences how well the body feels and how it responds to pressure. A cortisol deficiency may develop when your body is not producing the cortisol that it needs to generate during a workout.

4. Excess red blood cells.

The red blood cells in your body are responsible for using the oxygen your body needs. Sometimes you might have more red blood cells than is healthy. You would experience polycythemia as a result. This condition occurs when you have elevated levels of hematocrit and hemoglobin. Hematocrit is the ratio of the volume of red blood cells to the total volume of blood. Hemoglobin is a measure of the proteins needed for moving oxygen throughout the blood.

You may develop primary or secondary polycythemia. The primary form occurs when the red blood cells being produced within your body are developing and functioning incorrectly. This could cause sizable concerns in your body. Secondary polycythemia occurs due to erythropoiesis, a process where the red blood cells are produced within the bone marrow. The hormone erythropoietin is secreted by the kidneys with part of it being produced by the liver.

A blood test may be required to identify any of these problems that may cause issues in your body. You could potentially identify testosterone levels through some routines. A review of the red blood cells in your body may also be a factor that might be reviewed.

Chapter 10 – What an HGH Treatment Will Do For You (and What It Won't Do)

You may be surprised at how well an HGH treatment can restore your body's functions. You can control aging and many other problems in your life when you use a healthy HGH routine. You need to recognize that there are limitations to the effectiveness of HGH treatment as well as many benefits.

The Positives of HGH Treatment

1. Excess body fat can be reduced.

Aging can be noticed in many people who have excess fat. HGH helps you manage healthier metabolic routines, thus helping you to eliminate difficult fat deposits that you might have developed over time. This can especially be the case for controlling abdominal fats that are often hard to burn off. In fact, the reduction of abdominal fat is often found to be the most prominent sign that an HGH treatment is working as wanted.

2. You may develop added muscle mass.

HGH will help produce added muscle mass. You will feel less fatigue during a workout. This is also part of the reason so many athletes use HGH as a steroid of sorts. Non-athletes can benefit by using HGH to have stronger muscles.

3. Internal organs may become stronger.

Some organs might atrophy over time. These include organs that might not have the same capacities as what they used to have. You might not have as much lung capacity as what you used to have, for instance. Your heart might not be as strong as it used to be in younger years. HGH will help restore those organs to a healthier condition.

4. Skin will look younger.

The potential for your skin to wrinkle will be reduced thanks to an HGH treatment. New skin cells will reproduce more readily. The production of such skin cells is needed to keep your skin feeling and looking healthy.

5. Bone marrow cells will be produced easier.

You need healthy bone marrow cells to produce red blood cells. HGH assists in producing new bone marrow cells. These cells will respond by managing healthier bodily.

6. Your body will be at less risk of developing cardiovascular illnesses.

HGH improves your cholesterol profile. It should be easier for your body to control the development of unhealthy cholesterol deposits that may cause your arteries to clog and put you at risk of heart problems. You will be at a reduced risk of developing a stroke when you have enough HGH.

What HGH Treatment Won't Do

You may still be at risk of some health issues after you begin HGH treatments. Many of these factors relate to what has taken place within your body before the treatment began. This might require you to change some of your expectations.

1. HGH treatment will not reduce the effects of oxidation of your skin.

HGH is not going to reverse every wrinkle or spot on your body. The oxidation process can be intense and may be difficult to control or clear up on your own. It may be best to find a treatment sooner so you can keep the damages of oxidation from being any more intense than it needs to be.

2. HGH will not control the effects of other hormones.

The other hormones in your body will not be impacted by HGH. Added deficiencies in any other hormones might result in problems where the benefits of HGH will not be as strong as they should be.

3. HGH cannot reverse any of the proteins that were caused by excess glucose levels.

While you might help to reverse some of the signs of glucose levels being too high, that does not necessarily mean that you will immediately be healthier. Any proteins that were damaged due to high sugar or glucose levels will not be restored.

4. HGH will make your skin will look younger, but it will not erase all the damage.

You can use HGH to restore fresher look to your skin, but HGH will not eliminate all the damage that was caused by sunlight and other ultraviolet rays. The risk of your skin experiencing further damages over time should still be minimal.

5. HGH will not increase your lifespan.

While it is true that people who have HGH-related defects may have a slightly longer life expectancy after using HGH treatments, it does not mean that a person's lifespan will increase. The body can only live for so long. HGH just makes it easier for your body to handle more functions and to stay active for as long as possible. Your quality of life will improve, but you should not assume that HGH will make you live longer.

What is Hormone Replacement?

Hormone replacement might influence how well your body can manage its hormones and how your body might recover. In fact, the doctor that reviews your HGH profile and identifies what you can do for managing your HGH may suggest hormone replacement.

Hormone replacement therapy, or HRT, is often used to help those who are going through certain stresses and pressures within their bodies. This is especially true for women who are going through menopause. HRT may also be prescribed to men who are struggling with testosterone-related issues or those who are experiencing bone density loss. HGH treatments are often interpreted as being a part of the HRT spectrum.

HRT replaces the hormones that the body has lost. The process focuses on replacing what is lost with something new, particularly from synthetic or outside sources. An HRT doctor or specialist will be responsible for reviewing what you can use in the HRT process while also planning a program for managing the treatment process.

The use of HGH gel and other HGH-related treatments may be interpreted as a form of hormone replacement therapy. You can always talk with a doctor for more information on how an HGH treatment can work for you, but you should not assume that the process is going to be the cure-all that works for every single one of your problems.

Chapter 11 – The Hair and Skin Factor

HGH can be used to restore the health of your hair and make it look more attractive. Many people complain about how they are losing hair or that their hair is not as strong as it used to be. It is possible to re-grow your hair or to reduce the intensity of your hair being discolored over time.

In addition, you can use HGH to restore the look of your skin. While it is true that you might not repair some of the more intensive damages that have come about as a result of aging and other physical factors, you may find that HGH will do well for your body by keeping your hair and skin looking healthy.

Managing Your Hair

Hair loss and graying hair are among the most common issues that can happen with aging. Men are often more likely to develop hair loss, but women can also develop issues where their hair starts to thin and lose its strength.

HGH can counter the effects of DHT. Dihydrotestosterone is an androgenic hormone that causes baldness and graying hair. This can be found in older men for the most part, although women are often at risk of producing DHT. DHT causes hair follicles to shrink. This causes hair to stop growing. The hair that does return will become increasingly thinner. In addition, that hair will be lighter in color and lose its pigment.

The greatest concern about DHT is that it is much stronger than testosterone. The DHT will cause the hair loss to be more intense. DHT links to the same receptors as testosterone. The most important part of working with HGH with regards to DHT is that HGH will keep the DHT hormone from being as intense as it could be.

To get a better understanding of this, it helps to notice the three stages of hair growth. Your hair grows in the anagen phase, a process where the hair keeps on growing. This can last for a few years on average. The catagen process then takes place for a few weeks. This process allows hair follicles to stay renewed. The telogen stage occurs afterward for a few months where the follicles become dormant.

Naturally, you may consider adding a hair restoration medication to your routine just as well. Adding HGH may help you improve how that hair can return, but it might be best to avoid other hair restoration products when using HGH. You should use HGH first to see how well your body responds to the process. You can reduce the general effects of DHT when you use the right solution of HGH.

The effects of HGH on the hair are more prominent among men. However, women can expect to have their hair to look better too because split ends will be reduced. Their hair will also have a greater volume.

Working With Skin

Much has been discussed already how HGH can work to restore your skin's texture. There are many other things relating to your skin that should be noticed. The main reason why HGH is so useful is that it will help you with growing new skin cells. HGH will support renewing those skin cells to allow your skin to look brighter and more attractive. You will have clearer skin that is attractive and has a natural glow. HGH may also lighten some parts of the skin.

An excess amount of HGH can cause skin tags among other physical concerns and may make your body look less attractive. Your skin might become a little thicker. The threat associated with excess HGH totals can be significant.

Chapter 12 – HGH Self-Test

You might have to undergo an HGH self-test to determine how well your body is managing HGH and that you are getting the most out of your treatments. You can use the results of a self-test to decide if you need to speak with your doctor about a possible HGH gel treatment.

You might notice some significant signs in your body that suggest you are not getting enough HGH. These signs may be worse if you are older.

When to Self-Test

Your body will produce the most HGH when you are asleep. You need to get enough rest every night to help your body restore itself and to get the most out of its HGH. You might notice that a regular sleep cycle might not provide you with the healing or support you need. These could be signs that you are not getting the HGH you require.

You should also self-test based on any physical activities you do. Are you feeling a little more tired than usual during or after a workout? Are you struggling to get your weight under control? Maybe you are not able to work out as long as you used to.

The next section in this guide is about some of the things that you need to pay attention to as you're trying to make a self-test work for you.

Important Points to Note About Your Body

1. Review how well your skin is constructed.

You might notice that your skin is thinner than it used to be. The skin may not be as full as it used to be. You might notice wrinkling over time or even cases where the skin has become discolored. This could be a sign that there are not enough skin cells being restored.

2. Recognize how you are coping with menopause or andropause.

Women can suffer from menopause in their later years as the natural hormones being produced. Men can also experience a male equivalent to menopause called andropause. It is often hard to predict when these problems will happen in life. Menopause or andropause should be interpreted as a time where you need HGH support to restore how your hormones are functioning.

3. Your abdominal fat is growing in size.

Abdominal fat is notorious for being difficult to burn off and can develop primarily in middle age. Abdominal fat can be a sign of an excessive amount of insulin, but it may also be due to low hormonal growth. People who receive HGH treatments can experience an increase in insulin sensitivity while burning off more abdominal fat

4. You are consuming more alcohol than usual.

People often consume more alcohol as they age. Some people do this to forget about the difficult things that they are going through. Others might consume alcohol because they don't have much control over how their bodies feel. They might be at an elevated risk of muscular pain and stress. The addition of alcohol in the body helps to keep the pains from being prominent as alcohol is a depressant. Consider cutting down on alcohol consumption.

5. You are constantly waking up at night.

You already know that you might struggle to recover when you aren't getting enough sleep. Do you wake up at night and then struggle to get back to sleep? You may also notice that you are getting up between two and four in the morning; this could be a real problem that keeps you from getting back to sleep. Interrupted sleep disrupts your body's ability to stay healthy.

6. You are using corticosteroids more often.

Corticosteroids are medications responsible for controlling inflammation in the body. Hydrocortisone is the most prominent type of corticosteroid, although you can also find some that are stronger and only available by prescription. Prednisone and Rayos are among the most prominent prescriptions. These can become addictive if you use them too often and they might mask some of the pains in your body.

7. You are simply gaining weight.

You have to look at your general weight gain. People often gain a few pounds every year as our bodies store fats easier as we age. An HGH gel treatment may encourage weight loss that you might be struggling to lose on your own.

You should always talk with your doctor about any problems you are having. Going through a self-test can be the first step to decide if you have a problem.

Chapter 13 – The Basics of HGH Gel

HGH is available in many forms. You can find it through various injections and other treatments. You can't just take in oral medications for HGH as the oral compound would be quickly broken down by your body.

HGH is available in a gel form. This is one of the most intriguing ways how you can use HGH that may help you keep your body healthy. The gel product is easy to apply and can be spread over your body in a matter of moments.

The idea of using an HGH gel might sound unusual to some people. The HGH gel is topically applied to your skin. For instance, nicotine patches have often been used by people who need help control their smoking addictions. You might be surprised how well a topical treatment can work for your body. An HGH gel application can help you to get your body to feel better and be stronger.

Why Use a Gel?

The problem with many HGH injections is that they can be uncomfortable on your skin and cause irritation and soreness.

As well, the injection process is often not precise. You have to use an injection needle in a very specific spot on your skin. That needle has to be thin and fine enough to move through the skin easily and the needle has to be applied evenly and not at an angle. Any small change in how the application process works might be dangerous. You could experience irritation in the treated area. Some bleeding may also develop at the injection site. The frustrating process of mixing materials for injection can also be a burden. You might be at risk of mixing items incorrectly.

Working with a gel may be an easier option for you when aiming to make the most out of HGH. You can apply the gel on your skin without risking the material causing irritation or otherwise being difficult to add or move along your body.

The General Goal

HGH gel is designed to supply your body with a regular amount of HGH that you can utilize and feel comfortable with. You will have to make sure it is applied evenly and carefully for the best results.

HGH gel will provide you with a consistent amount of HGH. HGH levels can fluctuate in your body throughout the day and using the gel takes this into account.

Three Important Ingredients

Three particular ingredients are to be noted.

1. Glandula Suprarenalis Suis

The glandula is a reference to an endocrine or exocrine gland. For the sake of HGH gel, the glandula will be something that is similar to what you may find in the pituitary gland. The gel has been engineered to simulate the functionality of the gland responsible for the production of HGH.

The concentration of this ingredient is minimal. You can expect this to be about 10% of the formula. This is essentially used as a base for the gel.

Suprarenalis suis refers to the adrenal glands. These glands are responsible for producing adrenaline and steroids like aldosterone. The glands are found above the kidneys. The glands work with the growth hormone to facilitate how the compounds move through the body. It keeps the immune system from identifying the growth hormone you are absorbing as being a foreign entity that has to be removed. The protective nature of the hormone ensures that you will not be at risk of experiencing any significant problems.

2. Thyroidinum

You will require some form of thyroidinum in your medication. This is a part of the thyroid gland of a calf or another bovine source. It is a thyroid extract. Thyroidinum is used to manage thyroid-related issues and has, in fact, been used to treat various thyroid problems for many years. It is used to treat skin eruptions, a fever, pains around an impacted or treated area, or general aches, and pains.

3. HGH

The actual human growth hormone HGH is the main ingredient of the gel. Some HGH products contain as much HGH as two-thirds of the volume of the product. The total amount of HGH should be measured based on the concentration as different products have different concentrations of HGH.

What About Other Ingredients?

You may find some other ingredients to be of value to you in the HGH gel you use. These include purified water, which is needed to produce a firm base for the gel. This also allows the gel to be in a pump action container.

All other ingredients are inactive. This means that the ingredients are not going to influence your body. You can talk with your doctor for added details on how those specific ingredients might work for you. You can ask about any ingredients that you might be causing you concern.

Identified as Homeopathic

One thing you may notice about the HGH gel is that it is identified on the market as being homeopathic.

Homeopathy is treating a concern with small doses of something that would cause certain symptoms if used in large doses. This is otherwise known as the like-cures-like approach to handling illnesses and other physical concerns.

It is believed that providing the body with small amounts of the materials it might be impacted by will help to restore or trigger the natural healing process within the body.

Homeopathic treatments have long been prepared by mixing items like allergens and other things that weaken the body and diluting them with water or alcohol. It is believed by homeopaths that when the dosage of something is smaller, the healing process becomes a little easier to ignite. This is a part of why homeopathic treatments are used so often in the process of treating allergies.

In the case of HGH gel, the HGH being utilized is a minimal amount of what you are producing naturally. The HGH is not dangerous to your body, but having a small amount added through HGH gel helps to restore the natural functions of the body. This includes allowing for the natural production of HGH through the pituitary gland once again. Adding the HGH through the gel helps stimulate the body back into a regular routine.

Like anything else that works as a homeopathic product, HGH gel could be dangerous if you use too much. An excessive amount could be risky or harmful to your body. The excessive compound can trigger negative reactions in the body similar to what you are trying to control.

HGH gel can be a valuable solution for your restoration needs. However, as the next chapter shows, you'll need to look at where that gel is coming from.

Chapter 14 – How Does a Topical HGH Treatment Work?

HGH gel is designed to be a topical treatment. The HGH will be absorbed through your skin. The mechanism for how HGH gel works is something that should be reviewed.

Absorbed by the Skin

You will benefit from having a topical material as it provides you with better coverage over your skin than what you might get from a traditional medication. The gel works by moving through the body. As you apply the gel on the skin, the product will move into the deeper parts of the skin. The membranes in the skin will take in the compound to make it easier for the HGH to be processed. The material will eventually move into the bloodstream through the skin.

The main reason for using the skin is to target as many cells as possible that are responsible for healthy functions. Using the skin also lessens the chance of inflammation and irritation.

Targeting the Veins

You should add a medical topical material on the thinnest areas of the skin. The thinnest parts of the skin are normally where the veins are the most noticeable. These are the areas where a topical treatment will be absorbed by the skin and enter the bloodstream in the quickest way. It may also be easier for the application to dry up after a while. This should be comfortable and easy to incorporate into the treatment process.

What Makes the Gel Useful?

When looking at topical treatments, you will come across several choices. You might find basic creams that are an emulsion of oil and water designed to penetrate the outside layer of your skin. An ointment that is mostly oil may also work well. Transdermal patches are also noteworthy for how they release a drug within a certain amount of time with the skin absorbing the material and enabling the compound to move deep into the membranes.

A gel is a little different. A gel is much thicker in texture than a basic ointment or cream. Alcohol is often used as a solvent. A gel may liquefy at room temperature. A gel will adhere to the body quite well.

The gel is a self-drying compound. The consistency of the gel ensures that you will be able to administer it easily on your body without the material slipping or being too sticky.

Chapter 15 – Where Does the HGH Come From?

You might find plenty of HGH in your somatropin gel, but you might also be curious about where that HGH comes from. It is true that many HGH products are gathered from different physical sources. Somatropin can be collected from animal or human cadavers in many cases. However, some synthetic HGH compounds are available.

How Natural HGH Is Gathered

The earliest days of HGH production came in the mid-twentieth century when HGH would be gathered from human donors after their deaths. The process can be complicated and may be dangerous to the body and could entail some significant threats to the brain tissue.

In the 1950s, growth hormone was first gathered from human pituitary glands. The United States National Institutes of Health formed the National Pituitary Agency. The organization would work to collect and retrieve the pituitary glands of people who had died. The glands would be distributed to pediatric endocrinologists to treat children who were not getting enough growth hormone. The glands were able to produce enough HGH to help children to grow. The efforts in the United States spread to the United Kingdom, Canada, and many other countries.

As morbid as the process seems, it continues to be an interesting process to this day. Somatropin is still gathered through donor bodies to collect the natural growth hormone that is required. The extensive approach of filtering out the HGH can be complicated. The purification process has become more efficient, thus ensuring that the hormone that people need will be produced as required.

The effort involved with producing natural HGH is important and it is often difficult to collect HGH from living donors. The pituitary gland must be inspected to ensure that it is healthy and suitable for collecting the HGH. While some compounds from cadaver donors are still found on the market to this day, there are some products that come from a more modern form of gathering the material for use.

Producing rHGH

The product rHGH is a recombinant form of HGH. This is designed to use human genes that are added into bacteria and then used to produce unlimited amounts of the hormone. Specifically, recombinant DNA is used in the process as a bacterial solution will take in the DND to generate the hormone needed.

Recombinant DNA is a form of biology that has been in production since the 1970s. DNA molecules are collected and then replicated within certain organisms. The process is designed to create results that are identical to what people may find with other treatments. The rDNA has to be formed through a secure bacterial treatment that will allow for the production of the growth hormone.

The process for getting this DNA to produce new HGH was introduced in the 1980s, although it would take years of testing to see how well it would work. Eventually, this form of HGH has worked to help replace the use of cadaver donors, although the older process may still be noticed in some other parts of the world.

The most important part of using rHGH is that this is thought to be a little safer to use than other compounds. Much of this is thanks to rHGH not coming from any tissues that might have been diseased. By using rHGH, the HGH that is produced is safer for use.

Controlling the Risk of Creutzfeldt-Jakob Disease

Although the idea of creating HGH in this form might sound unusual, it is vital to control the risk of Creutzfeldt-Jakob disease, or CJD. This is a condition that has been linked to some people who have used HGH from cadaver sources. CJD is a degenerative brain disorder that can trigger memory problems and behavioral issues. Improperly formed proteins known as prions may cause the brain to stop functioning properly. The nerve cells eventually die, thus leading to tissue death.

Not all people who use HGH from cadavers will experience CJD. However, the risk is still something that many people are worried about and leads to efforts to avoid using this compound if possible. The threat involved can be significant. Using rHGH for treatments may keep that threat in check.

The Synthetic Consideration

The greatest worry that people have over rHGH is that while it can be a useful form of somatropin, not everyone will be happy about using it. The synthetic HGH may not be of the best quality when compared with real HGH. While the real compound might be pure, the risk associated with its use based on its source makes it a problem for some. Synthetic materials are not necessarily popular because people are still more interested in organic compounds. However, the synthetic version of somatropin is designed to be as functional and easy to handle as any other natural form. The use of actual DNA and proper bacteria for the development of HGH has made this useful. More importantly, the process of creating the product ensures that the supply will always be available.

The Development of Somatrem

One option you might consider for a synthetic form of HGH is somatrem. This is a little different from somatropin in that somatrem has an added amino acid. This is more of an anabolic material that will produce more side effects. The reason why somatrem is produced and used is that it is less expensive. This is in spite of the material not necessarily being as effective or useful as it should be. You'll have to be careful using it as it might produce more undesirable side effects when compared with a more traditional form of HGH.

Chapter 16 – How to Get a Prescription For HGH Gel

You will have to get a doctor's prescription for HGH gel due to the unique nature of HGH and how sensitive the material is. This is a hormone that has become very controversial and can be risky to handle.

The product may be abused by some people to increase their muscle mass. This has especially become controversial in many professional sporting competitions as people can use this to attempt to become more powerful and to have an advantage over the competition.

The best thing to do is to get a prescription from a doctor who is fully licensed to work with hormone therapy processes. A doctor who specializes in hormone replacement therapy will be easier to trust. That doctor can perform full tests on your HGH blood levels and can produce a hormone profile that identifies how your hormones are working. This may determine if the growth hormone in your body is what is causing your issues in life or if you have another concern that has to be resolved.

The most important thing about talking with a doctor is that he/she can help you find a real HGH supplement appropriate for you. Be wary of any product that you might find online that claims to contain growth hormone that you can get without a prescription as it is not going to be effective. That product might not contain any growth hormone at all.

Testing Is Required

The doctor you contact needs to complete a full set of tests and analysis of your body to see how you are managing your body functions.

The testing process should be thorough. The doctor should help you recognize what may work for when you. Testing is required to confirm your need for HGH as it is such a sensitive material that needs to be used properly.

Chapter 17 – How You Should Apply HGH Gel

You have to conserve the HGH that you take in, and you need to avoid adding more than necessary. The process of applying HGH gel is simple.

How Much Is Needed?

The HGH gel that you use should come in a bottle form. This would be provided to you through a pharmacy. A pump bottle is used to provide a consistent flow of HGH that can be applied on your body. This should give you a comfortable amount to apply without using more of it than necessary at a time.

You will have to use the HGH gel as follows:

1. Add one full pump of the HGH gel in the morning.
2. Apply another full pump in the evening.

This timeframe for applying HGH gel should help you get the right amount of coverage. This includes ensuring that the gel moves well over the body. You will have to allow time for the gel to be absorbed by your skin. The timeframe helps restore the HGH levels in your body throughout the day. This is especially important if your pituitary gland has been removed for any reason.

3. Make sure you use the HGH gel five days in a row.
4. Take two days off from using the HGH gel.

You cannot use the HGH gel too often and the two days off allows your body to rest. The potency of the material will be lost if you use too much and too often. More importantly, it will be easier for your body to use the material if applied within the correct timeframe.

5. You may consider adding two full pumps of HGH gel in the morning and again in the evening if handled well.

You might require two pumps of the HGH gel if necessary. This is for cases where you might not be getting a big enough response from one pump in the morning and night.

Where Is It Applied?

You'll have to apply the HGH gel to the right areas on your body. The key is to apply it to the thinner areas of the skin. These include areas where your veins may be noticeable. The application should be gentle. You can apply the HGH gel to the forearms, underarms, wrists, and behind the knees. These are the thinnest areas of your skin and therefore great places for you to apply the gel.

You should rotate the application spots as needed. Allowing a rotation of the areas should help you be comfortable without the body becoming too used to the application process.

The Main Benefit of the Administration Process

When you regularly use HGH gel, your body will metabolize the excess amounts of HGH. This should stimulate your body's natural production of HGH. The effort involved should help you to stay healthy while your body has an easier time with managing the HGH as needed.

After a while, it might be easier for you to use less HGH. You need to avoid using too much of this gel.

What About Storage?

Keep the HGH gel stored where moisture will not get be an issue. Allow the gel to stay in a dry spot so the material will not be affected.

Make sure the HGH gel is secured in a place where no one else can touch it. The HGH gel could be dangerous to other people. HGH gel can be risky for those who might not need it. This is especially the case when it comes to children. It is critical for any parent to ensure the gel is not accessed by a child.

Chapter 18 – The Use of HGH For Children

While most people know HGH as a material that may work for adult use, it can be used on children. There are many situations where children might not be growing as well as they should. This could be due to the body not producing enough HGH. A doctor can diagnose if a child is experiencing growth issues that may be caused by a lack of HGH. Proper treatments can help, but this would be on the advice and supervision of a doctor.

A child could be at risk of significant harm after using more HGH than what one really requires.

Common Causes and Signs of HGH Deficiency

A child could potentially develop growth hormone deficiency. This occurs when the pituitary gland is not producing the HGH that the child needs for regular health. The pituitary gland or hypothalamus may be damaged or might not have developed properly. The issue will prevent the body from being able to produce the growth hormone that the body requires. This deficiency is called hypopituitarism and is a congenital condition that a child is born with or could be an issue produced by an event that took place after birth. The acquired issue may be produced by a brain tumor, head trauma, an autoimmune condition, or other diseases or illnesses that directly influence the hypothalamus or other areas of the brain. Those who were treated for pediatric cancers, particularly around the brain, may also experience HGH deficiency due to the use of radiation for the treatment of various cancer forms.

The most noteworthy sign of an HGH deficiency is a child not growing at a particular rate. The regular rate of growth for a child should be consistent. The child should grow by 10 inches in the first year, 5 inches in the second year, 3.5 inches in the third year, and then about 2 to 3 inches a year onward to puberty. A doctor may analyze your child's height growth to see if there are concerns over how your child is growing. Any case where the child appears to be growing much slower than usual may be a sign of a deficiency.

There are many other concerns:

- The body's bone density mass will be decreased. This could place the body at risk of fractures.

- The body's cardiovascular health may not be as it should be. The body might not develop as well as it should due to critical tissues being abnormal.

- A child's energy levels may be limited.

- The child's facial features may appear younger than that of children who are of the same age. The bridge on the nose might not develop as well, for instance. Fat deposits may also be found around the face.

- Delayed puberty may occur. Some children with a lack of HGH will not go through puberty as others.

- The teeth are not developing as well as they should at this point.

- Hair is not growing as well. This includes hair around other parts of the body, particularly areas where hair should appear during puberty.

It should be noted that the condition does not impact the child's intelligence. The development of the brain should be normal.

However, a lack of HGH may cause impediment of a child's cognitive functions. The brain fog produced can be noticeable and may impair the child's ability to handle school studies.

The symptoms of a deficiency may be mistaken for other medical conditions. A doctor should be consulted to confirm a lack of HGH. The review of the child's body will be compared with regular development.

Is the Gel Appropriate For Children?

HGH products for children are available in oral vitamin forms and chewable tablets that are easy to process. Such items should be easy for a child to consume.

A gel may be used, but it is important for you to talk with your doctor about how it is used. You must review what the doctor prescribes for the child and then review how it will be applied. You'll need to keep the gel away from the child and ensure the gel is not easy to access. More importantly, you must ensure a proper routine is followed and that you monitor how well your child responds to the gel.

The specific amount of HGH needed should be smaller than what an adult would require. Talk with a doctor to understand the dosing of the gel.

What Inspires People to Get HGH Gel For Their Children?

You might not think that HGH gel is important for children to use. After all, there are times when a child might be growing and you might assume that the most growth will happen during puberty. There might be some signs over time where a child is not growing as well as you think.

HGH gel can help children who have experienced idiopathic short stature. This is a condition where the child is shorter than about 97% of other children of the same age. This might suggest the child might need to develop a little further, but in many cases, it might be a suggestion that the child's body is not developing properly.

Are There Risks Involved in Using HGH?

The greatest concern that parents have when it comes to HGH gel for their children is that the addition of HGH might be dangerous to the child. While it is true that HGH gel could help a child to grow to a regular height and to avoid any issues relating to the body's development, that does not necessarily mean that it is always safe. Granted, HGH gel can be risky for adults just as well. The risks that children might encounter can be significant and you should always follow a doctor's orders.

There is an increased risk of a child growing up and suffering a stroke following the use of HGH. This could be due to the brain developing quickly in the process. The brain might develop so as it may be difficult for the blood to flow into the brain properly. This could trigger a stroke in some cases.

The risk of bone cancer may also increase. While there are no guarantees that a child will experience such a problem, this could be a sizable risk that should be considered.

HGH may also increase a child's risk of developing type 2 diabetes. It is not fully clear as to why this would be the case, but it is assumed that type 2 diabetes is more prominent in those who experience sudden issues involved with developing excess body tissue. Watch for how your child's blood sugar levels might change following the use of HGH gel. You can use before and after tests to confirm that your child's HGH levels are suitable and safe.

The greatest risk involved might not be physical. HGH use might cause a child to think that there is definitely something wrong with being short. This could create a real problem as a child starts to think the wrong things about themselves and others.

A doctor will make the determination if your child may benefit by using HGH.

Chapter 19 – The Dangers of Excess HGH

You have to be cautious when getting HGH to work for you. The problem with HGH is that it can be risky and dangerous to take in if you are not careful with its use. There are several problems associated with excess HGH that could be significant.

An excessive amount of HGH is often referred to as acromegaly, which is how your pituitary gland produces an excess amount of HGH in adulthood. This condition is often caused by a tumor on the gland among other factors. Using more gel than needed can produce many of the effects relating to HGH and how it may function.

The signs of using more HGH than needed include the following:

1. Your body may experience some enlarged features that might be hard to control on their own.

Among the more common issues that your body might experience include issues like enlarged extremities, more distinguished facial features, and oily skin. Some skin tags may also develop around parts of the body. These outgrowths of tissue might protrude from the rest of your skin. Sometimes these tissues might expand to within the body and can cause difficulties with breathing, particularly during the evening hours. You may also develop a barrel chest, a condition where the chest size is much larger than usual.

2. Various organs may be enlarged.

The growth hormone might influence some organs. The heart, liver, spleen, kidneys, and other organs may be at risk of becoming enlarged due to the excessive HGH you use. This could cause those organs to stop functioning properly. The added stress on those tissues can be significant.

3. You may struggle to move your body.

Your joints and tissues may become enlarged and it may become difficult for you to move with ease. The risk can be significant and could negatively influence how well your body moves.

4. Heart-related illnesses may develop.

You may develop hypertension or high blood pressure due to the excess consumption of HGH. Cardiomyopathy, a condition where the heart is enlarged, may also be a threat. The condition causes the heart to work harder and you may experience intense fatigue. This can cause significant harm to your heart.

5. Your colon may develop polyps.

Polyps are growths that develop around the colon and can cause obstructions. Most polyps are noncancerous, although they might put you at risk of developing colon cancer or other types of cancers. The polyps can also block some of the functions in the colon and make it harder for the organ to stay functional.

6. Hypopituitarism may also develop.

The influence of excess HGH may cause your pituitary gland to stop functioning. This may cause issues where your body does not produce enough of the hormones required for staying active.

7. Sleep apnea can develop in some people.

Sleep apnea is a condition where you experience difficulty with breathing while you are asleep. The breathing issues you develop may come from your airways being obstructed. This would become significant as your tissues may develop and increase in volume. The threat may become significant as it can keep you from getting the sleep you require. This may also lead to some heart-related issues if the condition is not monitored or kept under control.

All of these threats associated with excessive amounts of HGH are to be observed as you go through an HGH treatment process. Be aware of how your body responds to HGH. Talk with your doctor if you ever experience any of these problems in your body. The key is to ensure that you are keeping your body under control and that you can avoid many of the heart-related concerns.

Always use HGH gel according to the instructions on the label and what your doctor tells you to do. Using the right amount of HGH prevents significant complications from developing and assists you in keeping your body in check without risking any issues.

Chapter 20 – What Is the Cost?

The expenses that come with HGH treatments can be cost-prohibitive. The cost may vary based on where you go and what you may find, but you can rest assured that HGH gel will cost less than what you'd spend on a more traditional solution.

Understanding the Expenses For Traditional Treatments

The greatest concern is that this can be very expensive for you to get. The problem with hormone replacement procedures is that they can be expensive. Fortunately, traditional HGH treatments are not as expensive as they have been in the past.

It used to be that HGH treatments would cost about $1,000 on average. This was for monthly procedures that would often be intensive. However, that total has dropped to $500 to $700 per session. This is obviously easier for you to handle, but you must notice how well the treatment can work for your body. Men often spend less on their treatments because they do not need as high of a dose of HGH as a woman might.

Many people find that the cost is worthwhile when the long-term benefits are considered. The potential for the body to feel younger and look better is something that all people like to experience. It often makes sense for people to spend a little extra on getting HGH treatments and avoid greater expense due to poor health.

How About a Gel Treatment?

The interesting thing about HGH gel is that it is much easier for your body to handle than many injections. HGH gel can be used without having to spend a lot of money in the process. You can expect various HGH gel products to cost about $50 to $150 on average. This would be enough for a month's use.

HGH gel will cost much less than what you might find for other treatments. The helpful and affordable nature of the HGH gel should help you stay confident in your ability to get the gel to work for you.

What About Insurance?

Many HGH gel products are not covered by insurance if they are only to be used for aesthetic needs and without any underlying medical issues in mind.

At the same time, there is a chance that your insurance might cover some of the cost associated with the HGH gel if your doctor prescribes a specific type of gel. The doctor should give a report on what you are using directly to your insurance company. The doctor will provide this information alongside your data to ensure the company knows you are using the HGH gel and that the costs involved will be covered. There might be limitations as to how much will be covered.

Contact your insurance company to see under what conditions they will cover the costs of HGH treatments.

A Final Note

HGH is a powerful compound that can help you build muscle mass and feel great. HGH is helpful for how it can help your body to grow and feel stronger. The best part of HGH is that it can help you to feel younger and to look your best. HGH gel can restore your cellular production and ensure your body won't struggle.

HGH gel is important to help you to look your best. Be aware of how HGH gel can work for your life and that you have a good plan in mind for making the most out of it. Don't forget to talk with your doctor about how HGH can work and what you can expect to get out of it for your health needs.

www.ingramcontent.com/pod-product-compliance
Lightning Source LLC
Chambersburg PA
CBHW071725020426
42333CB00017B/2391